Best Fastest Growing Vegetables & Fruit

For Home Garden

English Edition

by

Jannah Firdaus Mediapro

2021

While every precaution has been taken in the preparation of this book, the publisher assumes no responsibility for errors or omissions, or for damages resulting from the use of the information contained herein.

BEST FASTEST GROWING VEGETABLES & FRUIT FOR HOME GARDEN ENGLISH EDITION

First edition. March 28, 2021.

Copyright © 2021 Jannah Firdaus Mediapro.

Written by Jannah Firdaus Mediapro.

Table of Contents

Prolog 1

Best Fastest Growing Vegetables and Fruit: 2

1. Arugula 3

2. Spinach 5

3. Baby Carrots 7

4. Radishes 9

5. Cucumbers 11

6. Beets 13

7. Bush Beans 15

8. Bok Choy 17

9. Lettuce 19

10. Summer Squash & Zucchini..............................21

11. Okra 23

12. Kale/ Greens 25

13. Snow Peas...27

14. Broccoli 29

15. Green Onions 31

16. Turnips 33

Author Bio 35

Prolog

Would you like to grow a vegetable and fruit garden but feel like it just takes way too long? Well, the amazing thing is, it doesn't have to.

Instead, you can plant some faster-growing veggies and fruit plus have some great fresh green food options to choose from.

These vegetables and fruit can produce a harvest in as little as four weeks, and they give your family fresh greens to eat as you wait for the abundant harvest at the end of the growing season.

Best Fastest Growing Vegetables and Fruit:

Here are the faster vegetable and fruit options that you can grow in your small home garden:

1. Arugula

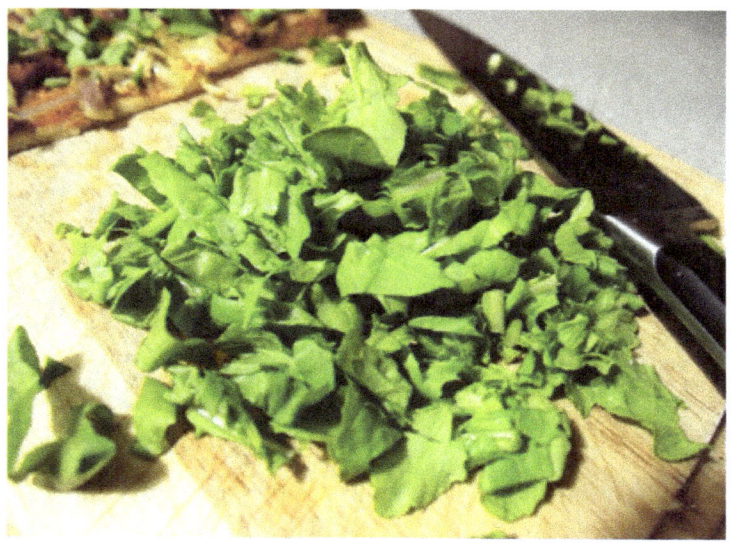

Arugula is a wonderful little green that has a peppery flavor to it. If you'd like to have a peppery green to toss in your salad, then you should consider growing this flavorful vegetable.

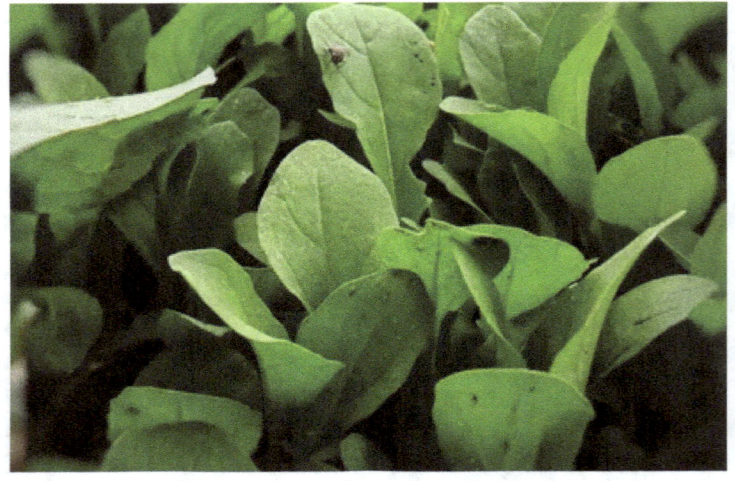

All you'll need to do is plant it, give it about a month to produce mature leaves, and then cut them when you're ready to enjoy. Then they'll continue to grow back each year for your enjoyment.

Arugula can be grown annually in nearly all zones and can be harvested after 30 days.

2. Spinach

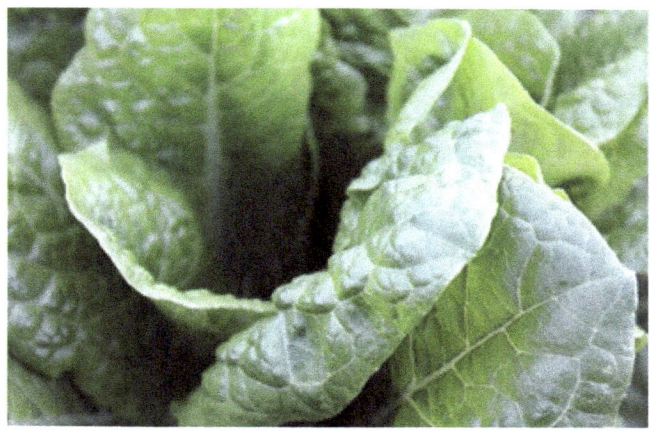

When you're looking for plants that add exceptional nutritional value to your garden, spinach is the answer to your dreams. Spinach is a source of vitamin K, vitamin A, vitamin C, folate, manganese, magnesium, iron, and vitamin B12.

Those are some real reasons why you need to grow spinach. Growing spinach can be a bit problematic if you don't have good quality dirt. You need to make sure you add plenty of compost to the soil. After you plant spinach, it's ready to harvest in 4-6 weeks.

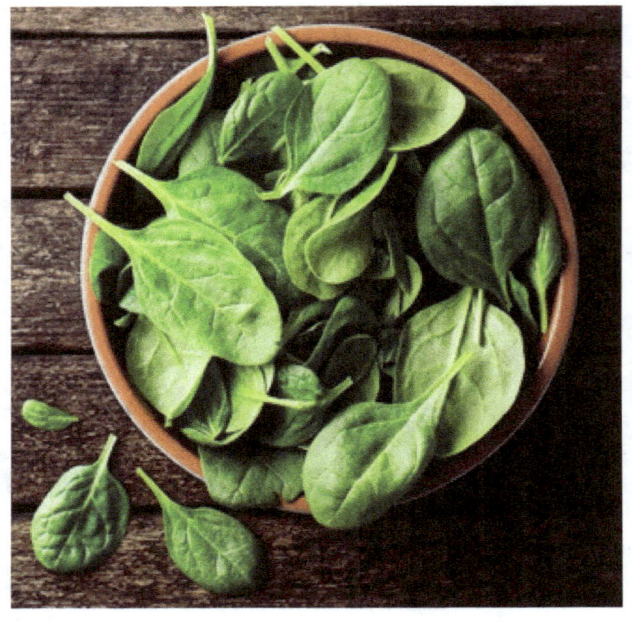

Spinach is frost-hardy, so you can sow it in the garden 2-3 weeks before the final frost date. Spinach can be a nice addition to any salad, or you could prepare the spinach fresh like in this recipe.

Spinach can be grown in Zones 3-9, and the leaves can already be harvested 6 weeks after planting.

3. Baby Carrots

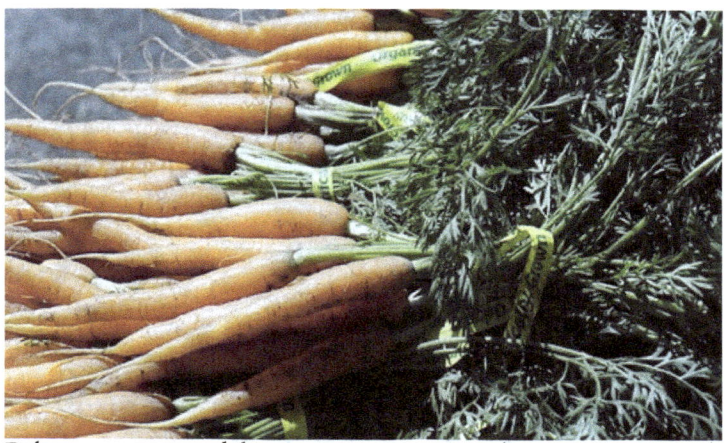

Baby carrots taste delicious, are a great snack, are great to cook with, and don't take as long as full-sized carrots because they don't have to grow to be as large.

So if you enjoy carrots and want them quickly, then you'll definitely want to pick the baby carrot variety. Plant them in the ground, or in a container garden for versatility.

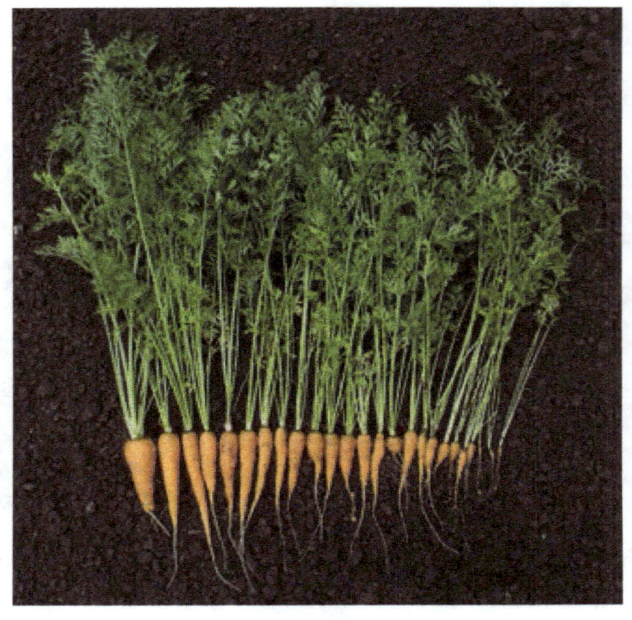

Either way, be sure to directly sow the seeds in quality dirt. Then in about 30 days, you'll have your first harvest.

Baby carrots can be grown in zones 4-10 and can be ready within a month from sowing.

4. Radishes

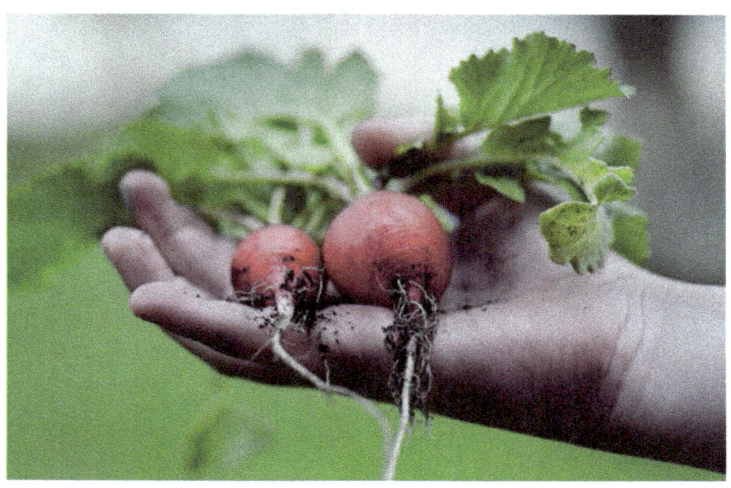

Radishes are probably one of the fastest plants you can grow. They are also super simple to grow as well.

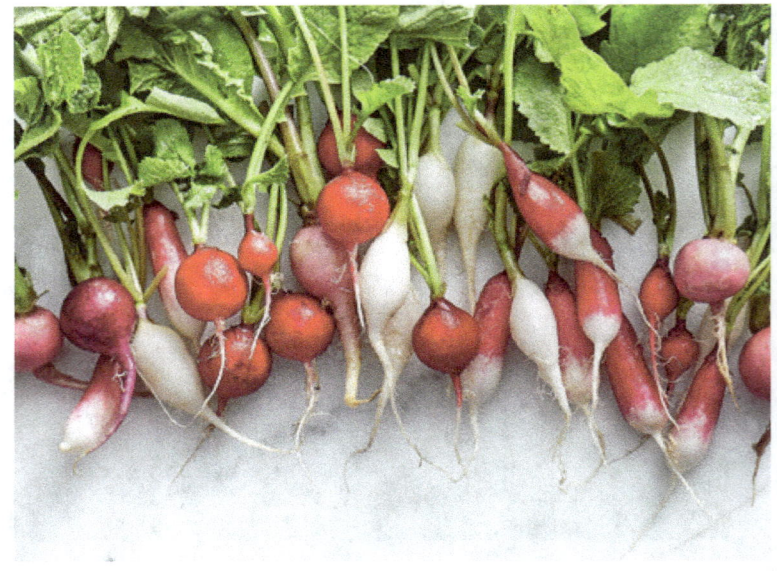

If you'd like to try and grow your own vegetables, radishes are excellent fast-growing vegetables to start with. You'll directly sow these seeds in quality soil.

Radishes can be harvested in about 22-50 days and can be grown in zones 2-10.

5. Cucumbers

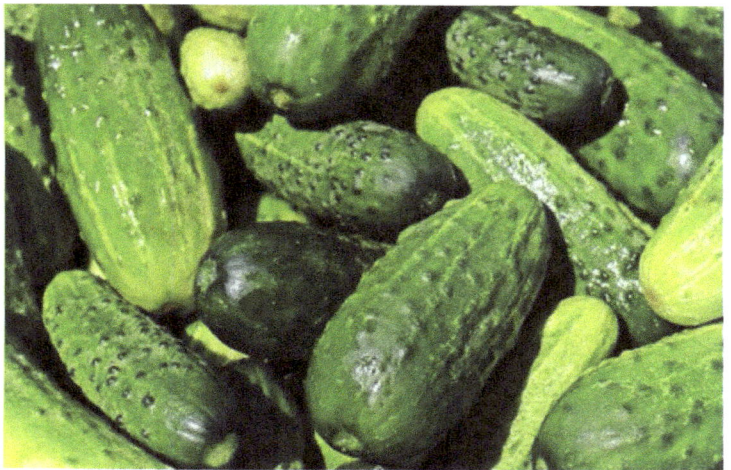

Cucumbers are a very versatile plant to grow. You can make lots of delicious recipes with them. You can start with eating them fresh.

Then they could be a great addition to a salad. When you are "cucumbered out", you can start making pickles with the fresh cucumbers.

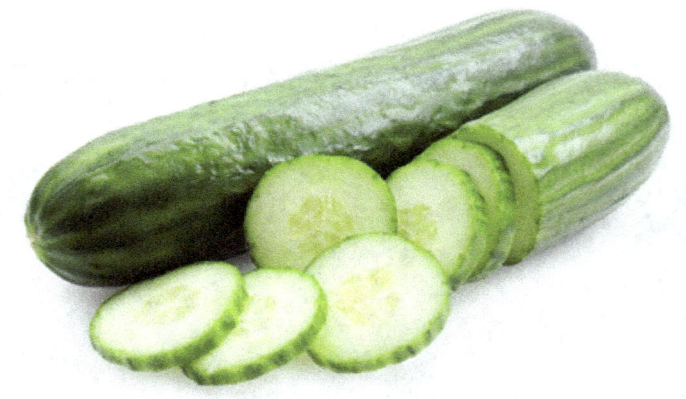

But be advised that cucumbers like to run so you'll need to either place them on a trellis or give them plenty of space to grow.

Cucumbers can be grown in zones 4-11 and if you want to make pickles the baby cucumbers can be harvested as early as 50 days after planting.

6. Beets

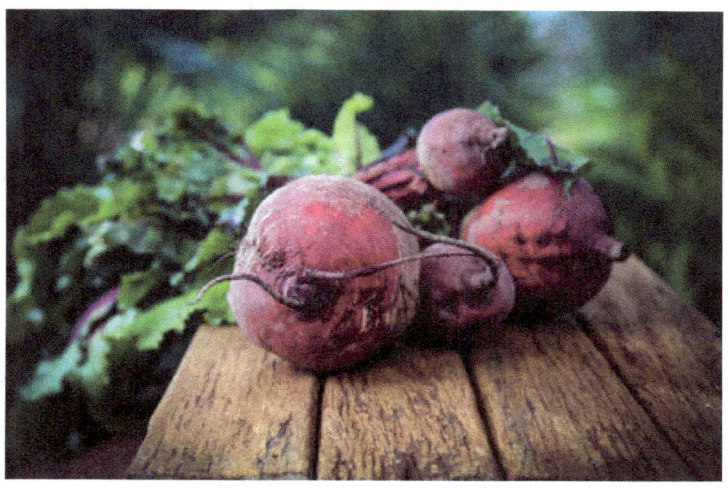

Beets are one of those vegetables that you either like or you don't. But even if you don't like the actual beet itself, you may enjoy the greens that come from the plant.

So either way, it is a great vegetable to grow if you'd like to have a harvest in a hurry. It is good to grow in the spring or when we are heading into fall because they can withstand a little heat, but don't like the super-hot temperatures we often experience during summer.

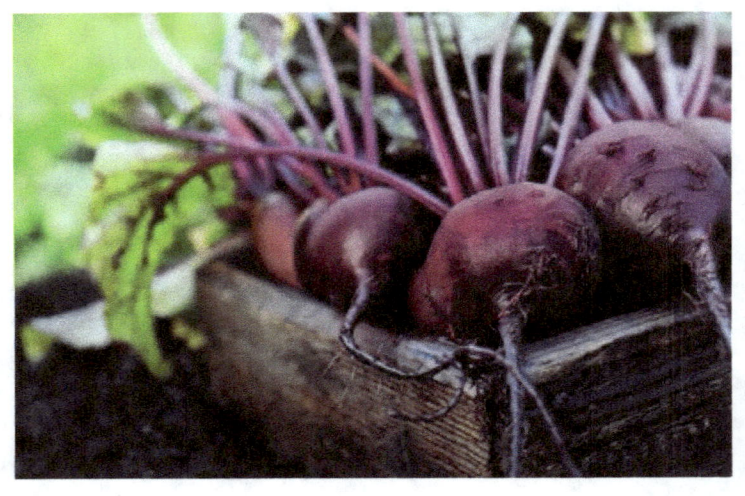

Beets can be harvested in around 50 days, however, the greens can be harvested from 30 days. They grow well in zones 2-10.

7. Bush Beans

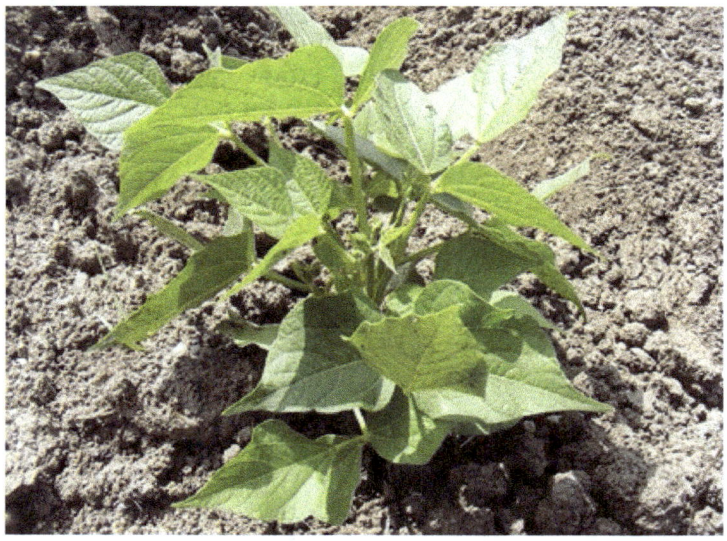

Bush beans are my favorite kind of bean. They grow beautifully in the garden, they are easier to prepare when canning green beans, and they also produce a quicker harvest.

So if you love tender green beans, then consider planting a bush bean variety. All you'll need to do is directly sow the seeds into quality dirt.

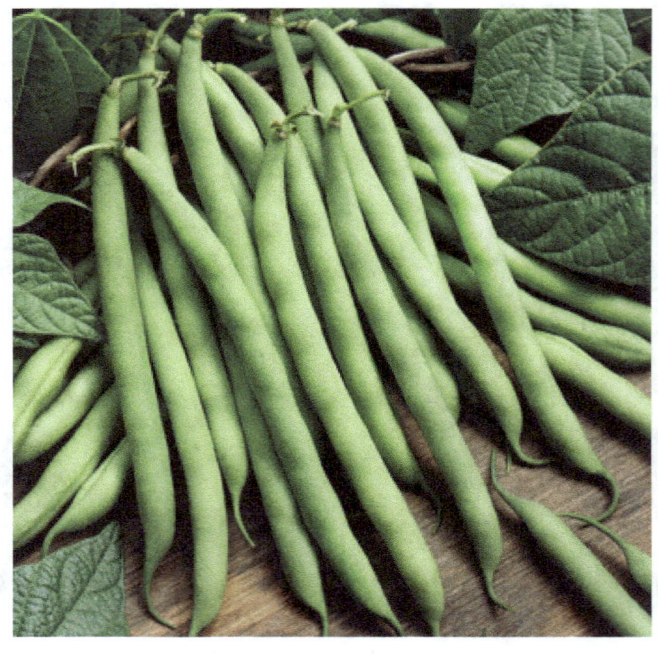

Then over time, with water and sunlight, they will produce a beautiful green bean bush.

Bush beans will be ready in around 40-65 days and grow well in zones 3-10.

8. Bok Choy

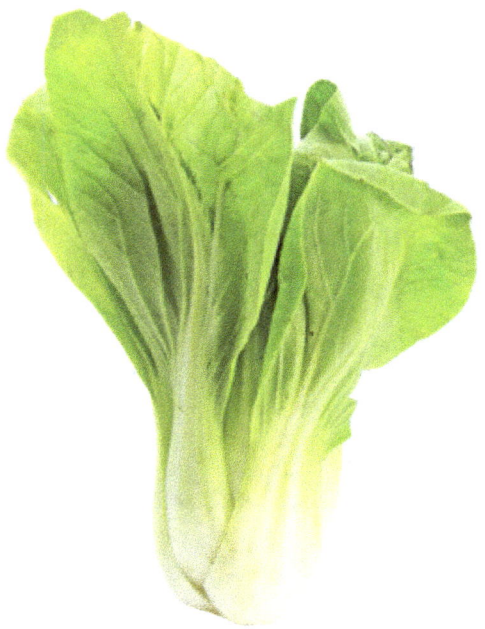

Bok Choy is a fun plant. It looks fun, and it is even fun to say its name.

But it is also a great plant to grow because it can produce a mature harvest in around 30 days. If that isn't a super-fast plant, I'm not sure what is.

If you are looking for something different to grow that will produce a fast harvest, then you should definitely consider Bok Choy.

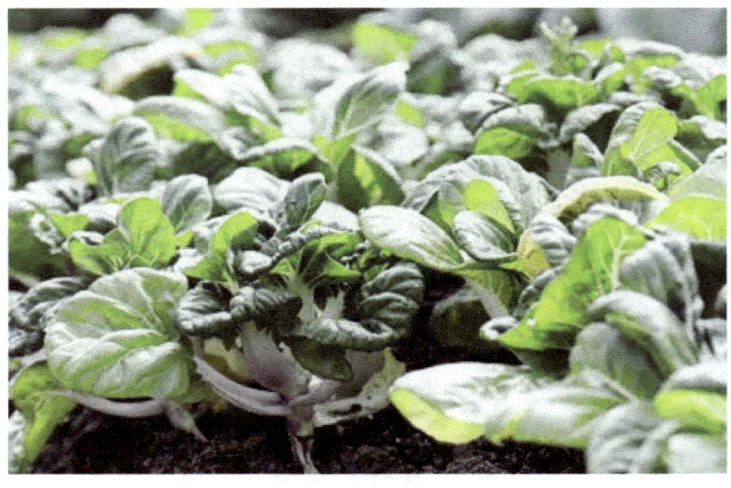

Bok Choy grows well in zones 4-7 and individual leaves can be harvested after 21 days, or the whole he

9. Lettuce

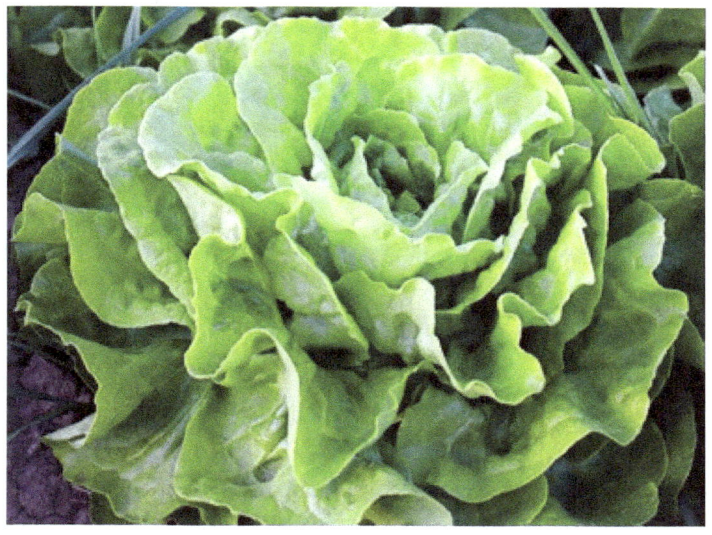

Lettuce is such a versatile plant. There are so many different varieties to choose from that you can have a different flavor and crunch with each one.

But the great thing about lettuce is that it is hearty so it can grow in colder temperatures, and it also doesn't take very long to produce a mature harvest.

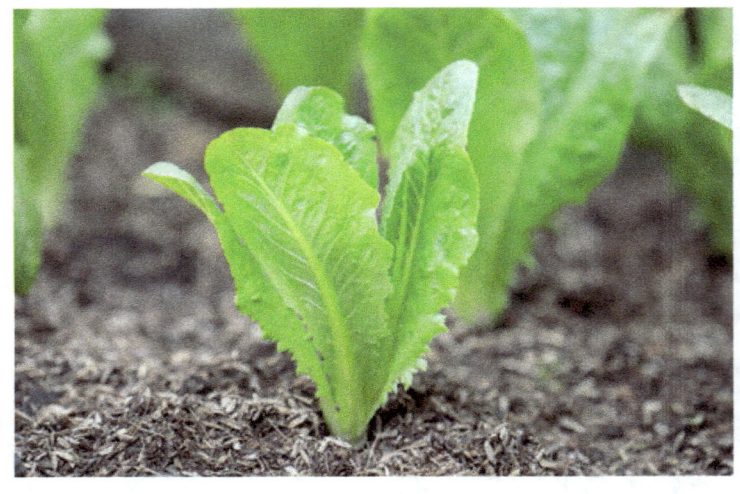

If you want something healthy, green, and fast, then you should definitely consider planting lettuce.

Depending on the Lettuce variety, harvest can be about 30-60 days after planting, ideally in zones 4-9.

10. Summer Squash & Zucchini

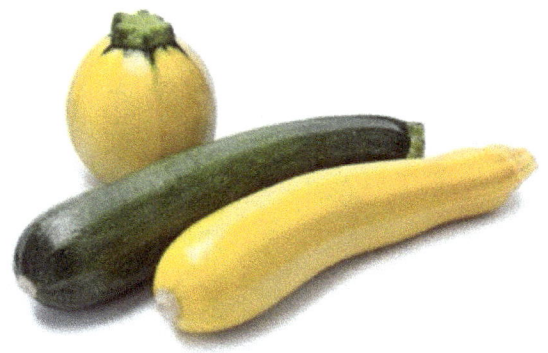

Summer squash is probably one of my favorite vegetables to enjoy during the warmer months. It tastes delicious, is easy to grow, and produces quickly too.

So if you need to learn how to grow your own squash, here is a great resource to help you along the way.

But a quick overview is basically, you directly sow the seeds in quality soil, water them, and wait for them to grow and produce.

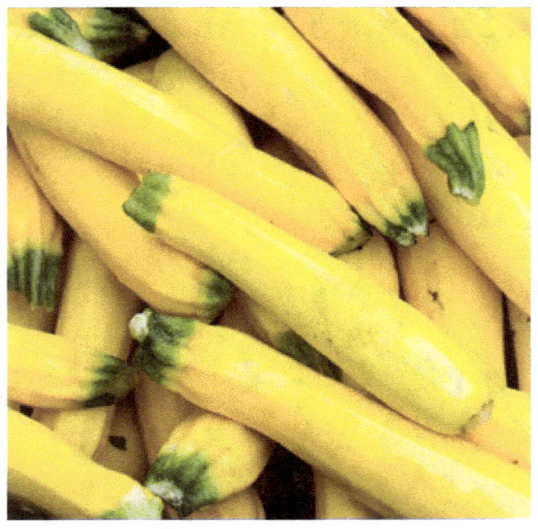

However, you'll want to be sure to harvest your squash or zucchini when they are young for better flavor.

Zucchini, a Summer Squash variety, grows best in zones 3-10 and can be harvested almost daily

11. Okra

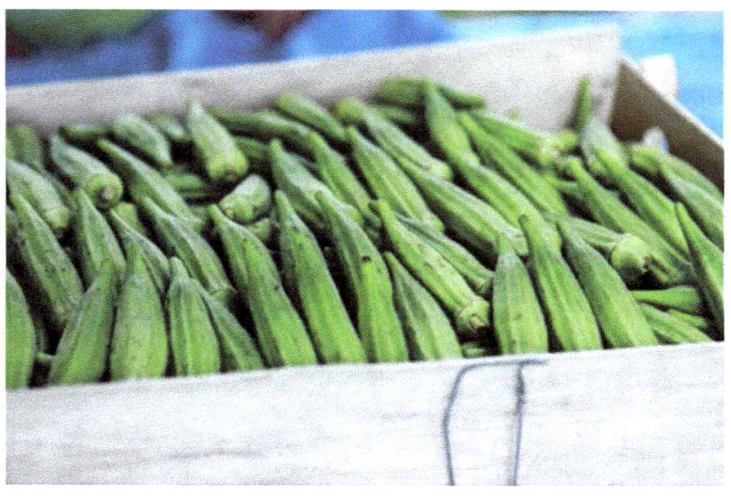

Okra is another favorite vegetable of mine. It only takes about 50 days to produce a mature harvest.

Then you are clear to pick it and fry it up into a delicious side dish that many enjoy.

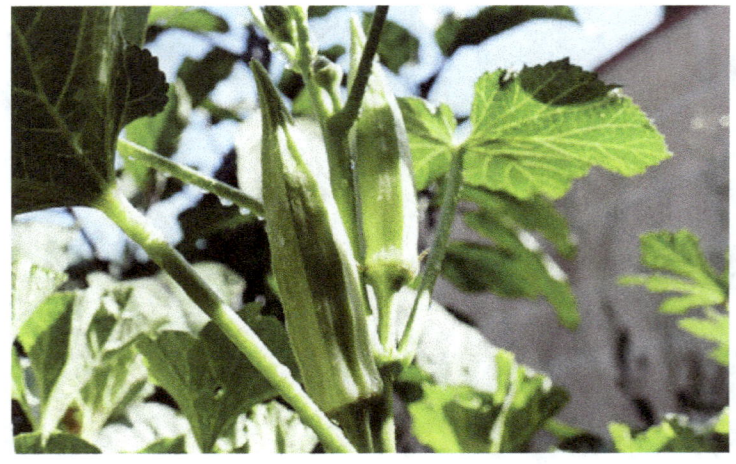

But you can also prepare okra in other ways as well. Go ahead and enjoy this fast-growing vegetable. You'll be glad you tried it!

Okra can be planted in zones 3-9 and the Cajun Delight variety matures in 50-55 days after planting.

12. Kale/ Greens

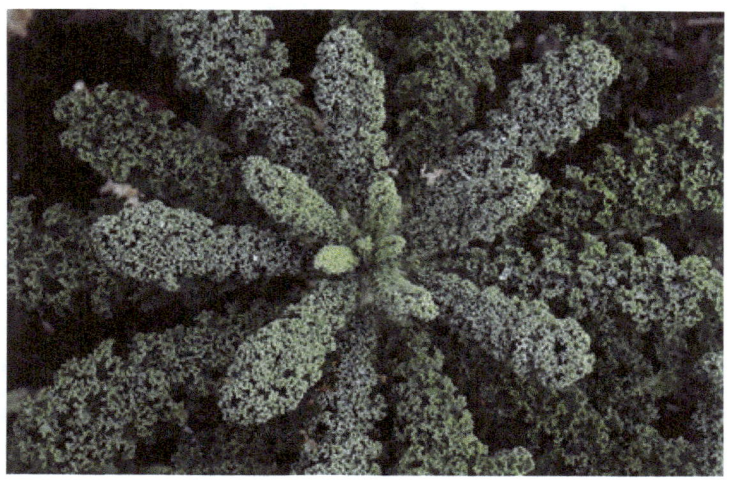

I am a huge fan of greens and kale, but it has not always been that way. In fact, growing up, I wouldn't touch them with a ten-foot pole.

But I've learned it is all in the preparation. I think I also love them even more now because I try to grow most of my family's food.

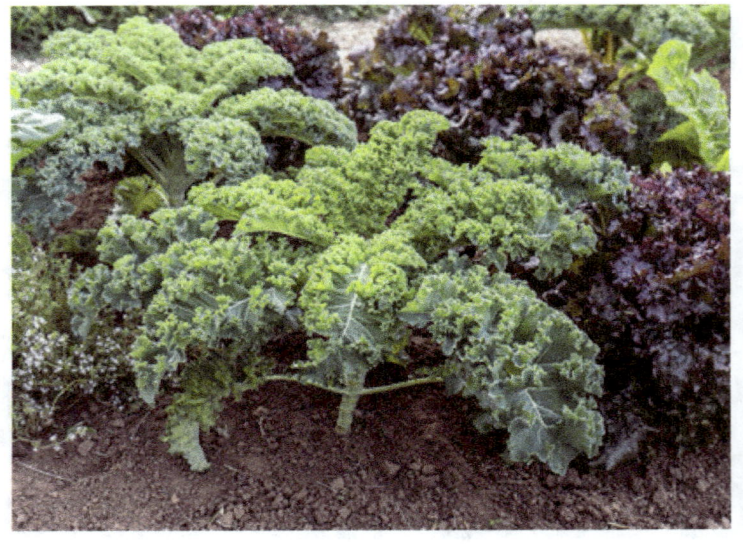

And who doesn't love a vegetable that is fast to produce? You can pick baby greens from kale or mustard greens in only 25 days.

Then you can have your mature leaves in about 50-65 days.

Kale does well in cold and can be grown in zones 8-10 all year round, but can also be planted in zone 7.

13. Snow Peas

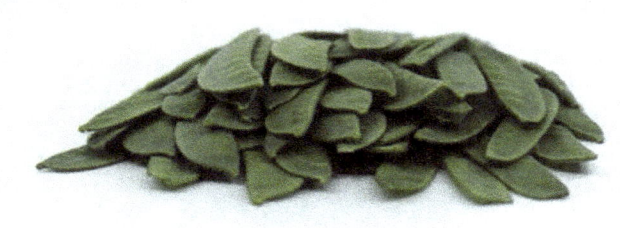

Peas have always been interesting to grow to me. In my experience, you have to plant a lot of them to get a decent harvest.

Now, for me when I say decent, I mean enough to eat and preserve.

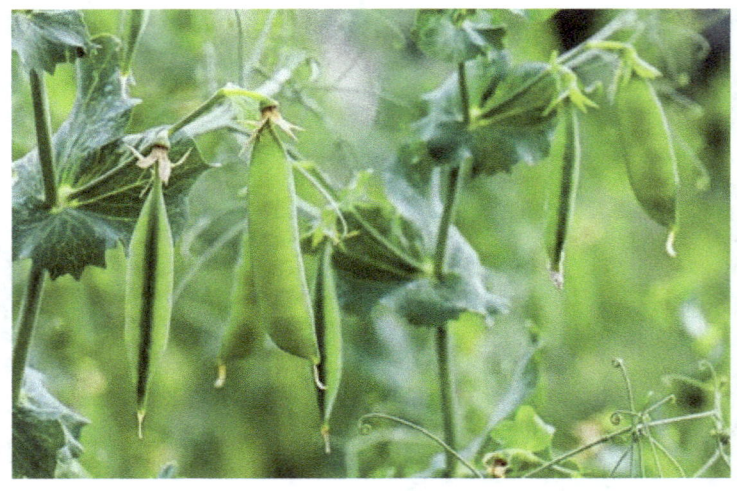

But if you just like to plant something to eat on it, then this could still be a good option for you. Snow peas take around 10 days to complete the germination process.

Snow peas can be harvested at around 60 days. They do well in zones 3-11.

14. Broccoli

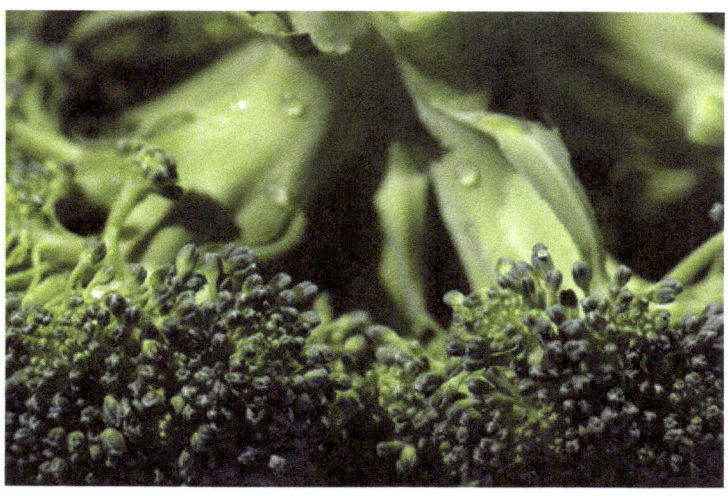

I love broccoli. As a kid, it fascinated me because it looked like tiny trees. As an adult, I love it because I can put cheese on it, butter on it, or seasonings and enjoy it again and again.

But as someone that tries to produce most of their own food, I love broccoli because it likes colder weather. It is refreshing to be able to grow something green when the temperatures are still nippy outside.

So if you love broccoli too, then know that you can grow it and have it ready for harvest in around 60 days. That is how long it takes for it to make mature heads.

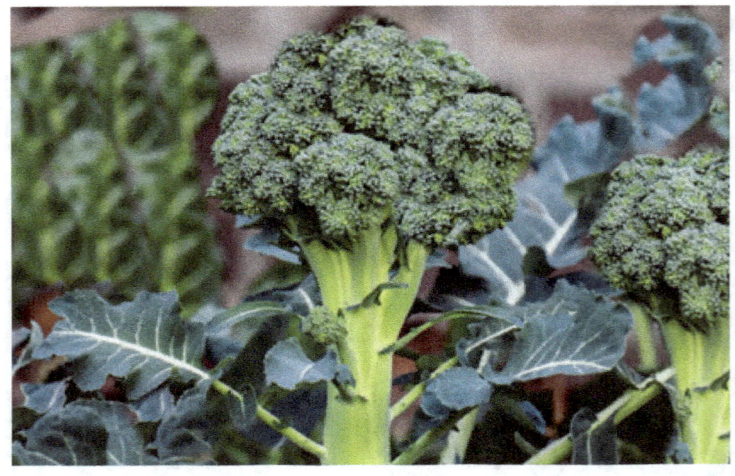

However, you could enjoy smaller heads of broccoli even sooner than that. It is all about your preference.

Grown in zones 3-10, Broccoli can be harvested after day 58, depending on the variety.

15. Green Onions

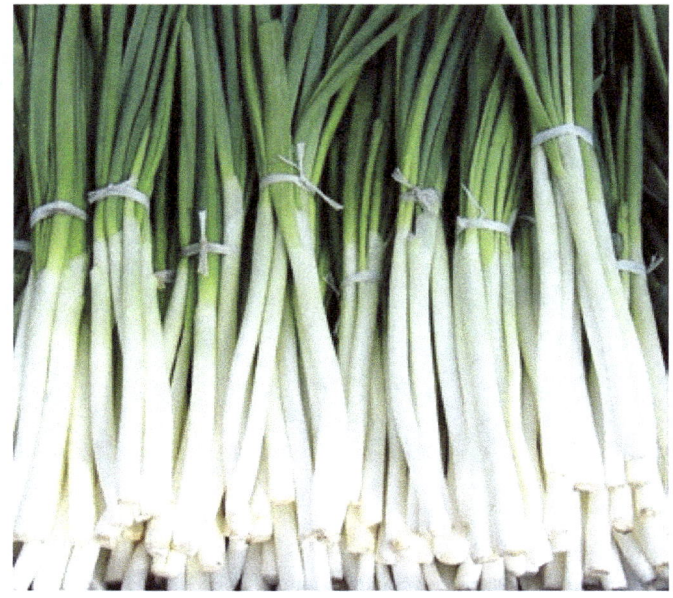

Green onions are another really versatile plant. You plant onions as bulbs. The bulbs take around 6 months to produce full-size onions.

But you can get green onion stalks at around 3-4 weeks. They taste delicious as a garnish for soups or to be added to stir-fry as well.

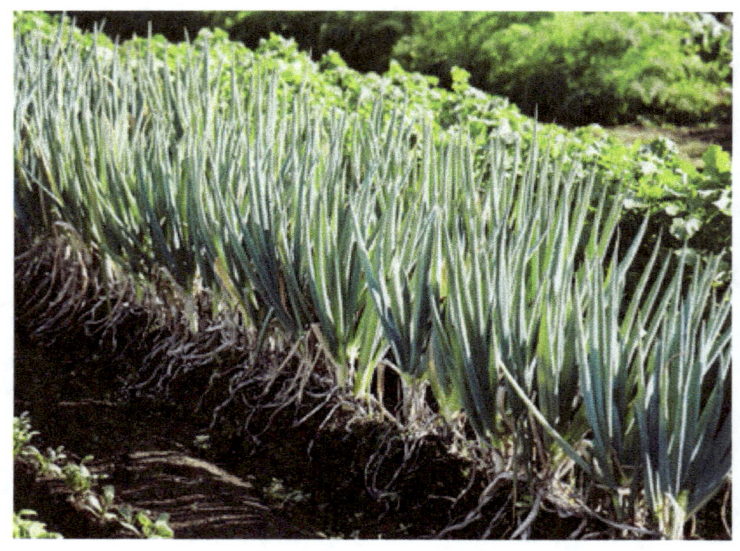

So if you want something green, fresh, and packed with onion flavor, then know that you can have all of that in less than a month.

Green onions grow in zones 3-9 and can be ready in 20-30 days from planting.

16. Turnips

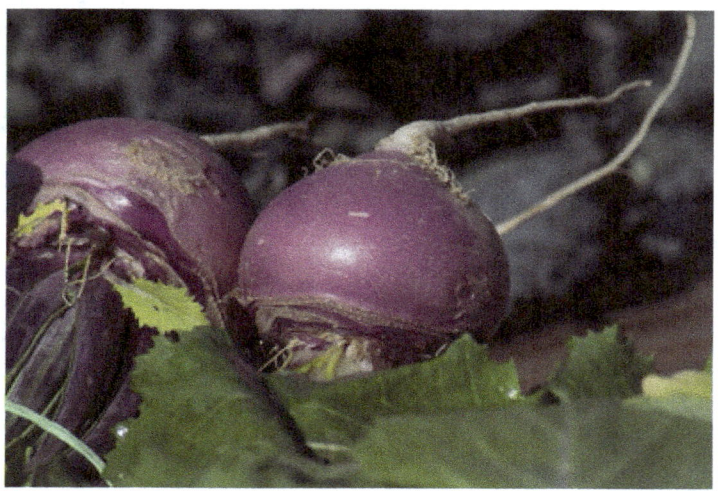

Last but not least, Turnips are another vegetable that is amazing because you get two products in one plant. Turnips produce a bulb that has a very unique flavor. Turnips are loaded with fiber, vitamin A, vitamin C, and folate, along with minerals such as calcium, magnesium, iron, and protein.

That's a serious reason to stick these into your garden. Turnip greens are ready to eat in 40 days, but the turnip bulbs take about 60 days to mature. You might be apprehensive about eating turnip greens, but they're particularly delicious.

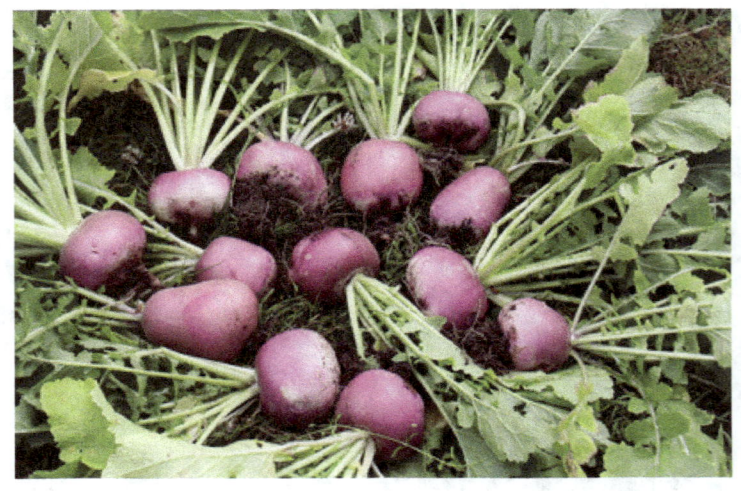

So if this sounds good, then know that you can have turnip greens in 40 days and turnip roots in around 60 days.

Turnip varieties such as the Market Express can be ready in as little as 30 days, and Turnips do well in zones 3-9.

Author Bio

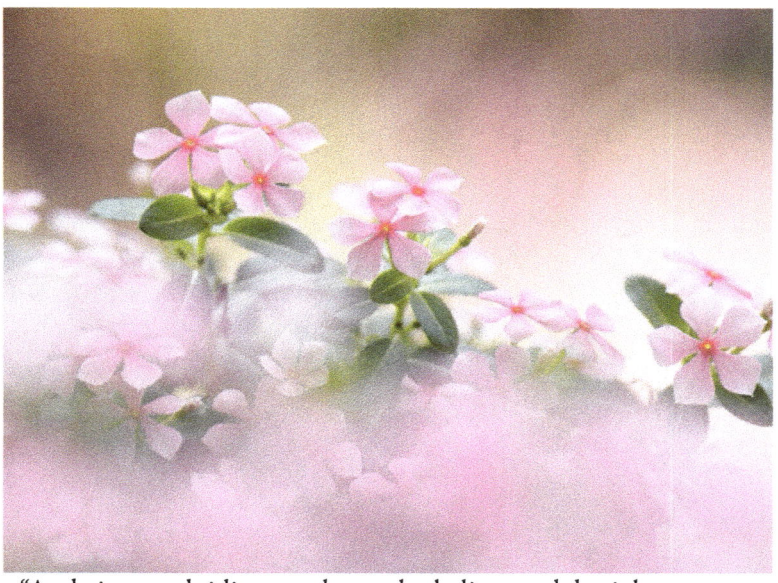

"And give good tidings to those who believe and do righteous deeds that they will have gardens [in Jannah Paradise] beneath which rivers flow.

Whenever they are provided with a provision of fruit therefrom, they will say, 'This is what we were provided with before.' And it is given to them in likeness.

And they will have therein purified spouses, and they will abide therein eternally."

(The Noble Quran 2:25)

www.ingramcontent.com/pod-product-compliance
Lightning Source LLC
LaVergne TN
LVHW021951060526
838200LV00043B/1969